Made in United States
North Haven, CT
15 December 2022

29125562R00057